My Grandma's Hip Replacement

A Children's Educational Book on Total Hip Replacement

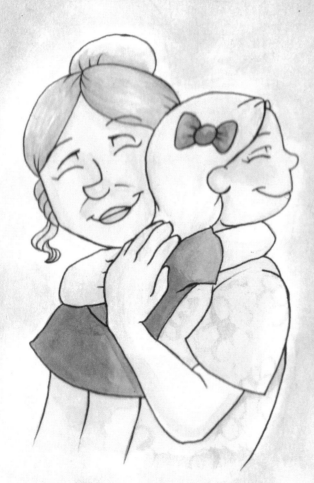

By Kendall Slutzky

Illustrated by Hannah Warner

AuthorHouse™
1663 Liberty Drive
Bloomington, IN 47403
www.authorhouse.com
Phone: 1-800-839-8640

First published by AuthorHouse 1/26/2010

ISBN: 978-1-4490-6631-4 (sc)

Library of Congress Control Number: 2009913917

Printed in the United States of America
Bloomington, Indiana

This book is printed on acid-free paper.

authorHOUSE®

Author Dedication:

To my two beautiful daughters, Taylor Ashley and Jordan Paige, for giving me the desire to educate them in my and their grandfather's field of work of total joint replacements.

To my husband, Michael: thank you for all of your support-I love you.

To Operation Walk:

May this organization continue to grow and prosper with proceeds from this book.

(please see description on the next page)

Operation Walk

Imagine being confined to a wheelchair or a lifetime of crutches as a result of disabling pain from joints destroyed by arthritis. The intense, never-ending pain that patients such as these endure makes conducting normal, productive lives difficult to impossible. For these people, even the most basic everyday activities, such as moving across a room or getting in and out of a chair, are difficult tasks. Because of their inability to walk and provide for themselves, many lose their jobs, their families, and the ability to experience the basic joys of life.

Imagine further the dream of suddenly being able to walk again free of pain. It is the goal of Operation Walk to fulfill this dream for those with little or no access to life-improving care. Operation Walk is a not-for-profit, volunteer medical service organization that provides free joint replacement surgery for patients in developing countries (and occasionally in the United States) who have debilitating arthritis or other bone and joint conditions.

Initially founded in Los Angeles, California, in 1994 by orthopedic surgeon Lawrence D. Dorr, MD, Operation Walk has grown to incorporate more than ten chapters throughout the U.S. and Canada. Since its inception, the numerous chapters of Operation Walk have traveled to multiple continents and have successfully helped hundreds of people regain the joy of walking.

The mission trips are designed to restore the gift of walking to as many people as possible. With sixty to eighty joint replacement procedures typically performed by the surgeons during each mission trip, the Operation Walk surgeons and volunteers simultaneously educate local healthcare workers in advanced surgical and rehabilitation techniques. Operation Walk relies on the generosity of donors to help fund each mission trip. Without these donations, it would be impossible to do this amazing work and fulfill the vision of changing people's lives by restoring the gift of walking.

www.operationwalk.org

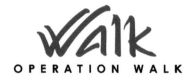

OPERATION WALK

"Taylor, we are going to go see Grandma today," said Mommy. "She is at the <u>hospital</u>. A hospital is where people go to get better when they have boo boos or are sick."

"Why is she at the hospital?" asked Taylor.

"Grandma has a boo-boo on her hip. She had what is called a <u>total hip replacement</u>."

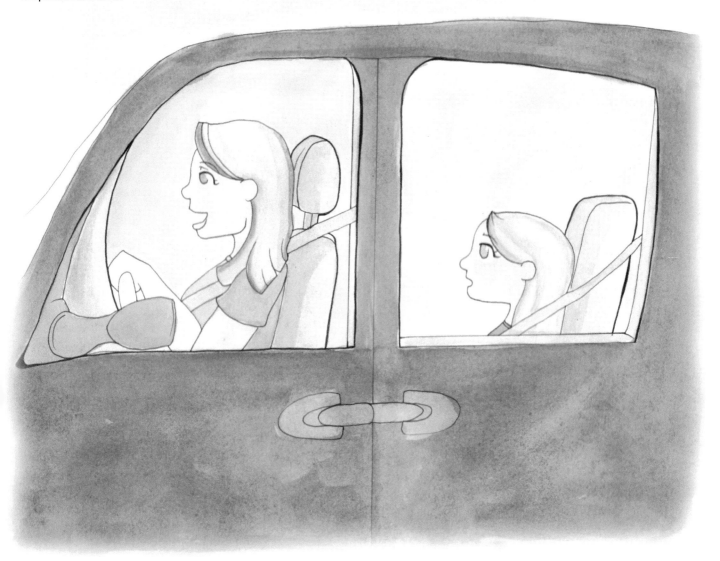

As Taylor and Mommy arrived at the hospital, they got on the elevator to go up to the fourth floor, where Grandma was being cared for. Taylor knocked on the door to her room and saw Grandma lying on the hospital bed and Grandpa standing next to her. Taylor looked at Grandma and was a little unsure about what was going on.

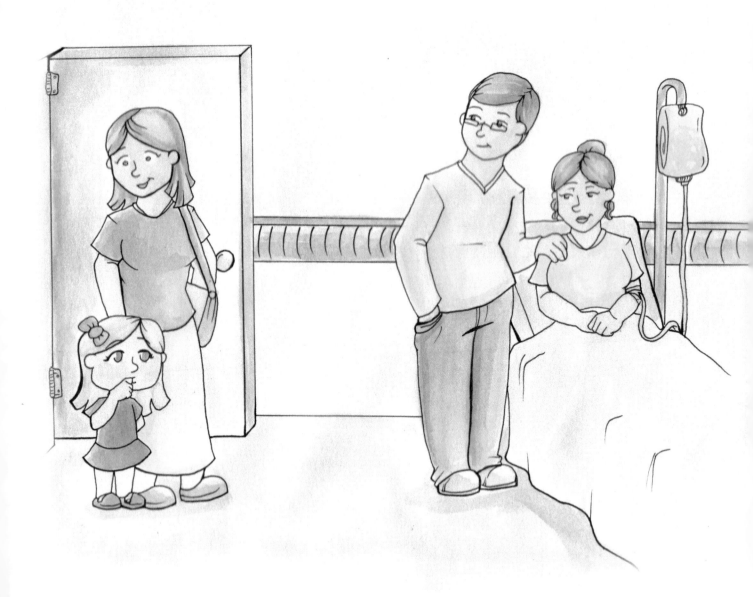

"Hi Taylor!" said Grandma, who was very happy to see her.

"Hi Grandma! I have missed you bunches and bunches!" said Taylor.

"I missed you too," said Grandma. "I am so glad you came to the hospital to see me. You made my day!"

Taylor, who was still a little unsure of what was going on, asked, "Grandma, what are all of those strings that are attached to you?"

"Those are not strings. They are tubes attached to my body that give me medicine to make me feel better. This is what you call an <u>IV</u>. When I go home, they will take the tubes away."

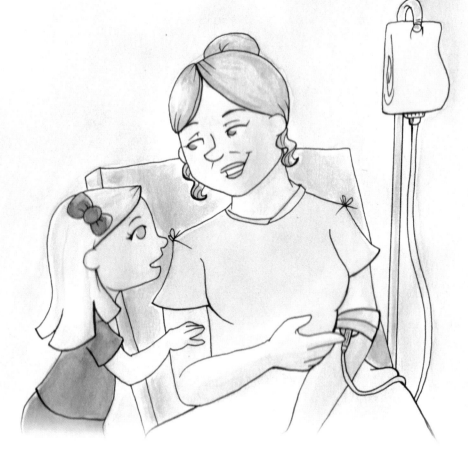

"Why do you need medicine, Grandma?" asked Taylor. "Do you have a cold?"

"No, sweetheart. I just had <u>surgery</u> on my hip, and the medicine will make my hip feel better.

"What is surgery, Grandma?"

"There are many kinds of surgery. In my type of surgery, the doctor took out my old hip bone that hurt a lot and gave me a new one that won't hurt after it has healed. It is called a total hip replacement."

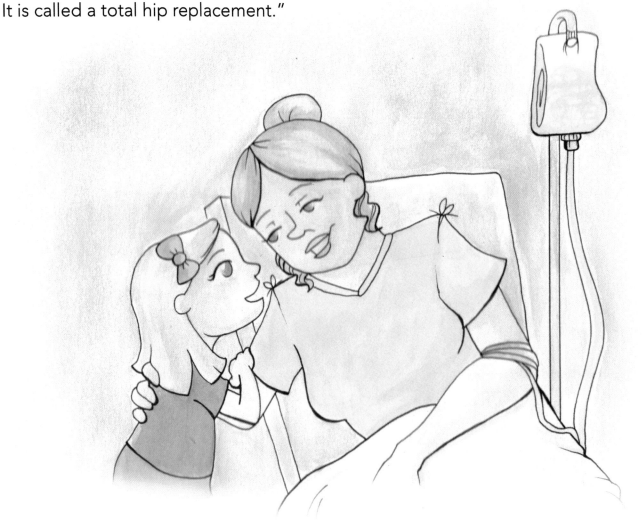

"Then I stay in the hospital for about two to three days, and the <u>doctors</u> and <u>nurses</u> take care of me until I can go home," explained Grandma. "Look, here comes one of my nurses. Her name is Ashley, just like your middle name!"

"Well, look who came to visit!" said Ashley, the nurse. "What is your name?"

"Taylor; T-A-Y-L-O-R!" said Taylor.

"What a pretty name!" said Ashley. "That is so wonderful how you can spell your name! My name is Ashley. It is so nice to meet you! Your grandma is doing great! She will be able to come home and play with you really soon."

"I hope so; I miss her so much!" said Taylor.

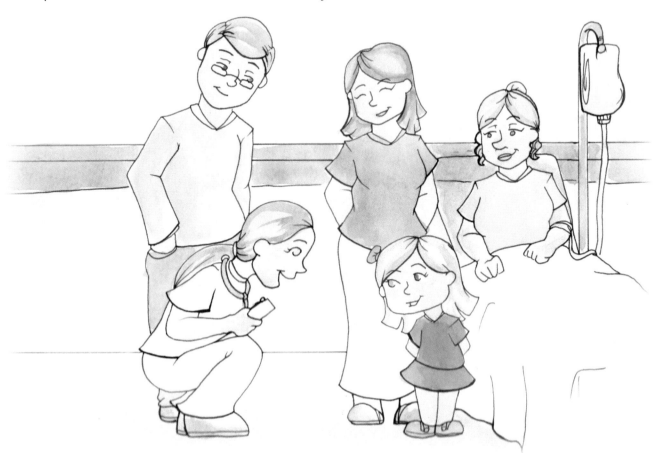

"Would you like to see my boo-boo?" said Grandma. "Ashley is going to change my <u>bandage</u>."

"Yes! Is it like the boo-boo on my elbow from when I fell the other day?

"No, not quite, sweet girl. However, both boo-boos will get better—just at different times."

"I want to see it, Grandma," begged Taylor.

Ashley took off the bandage so Taylor could see the boo-boo.

"What is that?" Taylor said with surprise, looking at Grandma's hip.

"This is called my <u>incision.</u> It is where the doctor cut through my skin to put in my new hip."

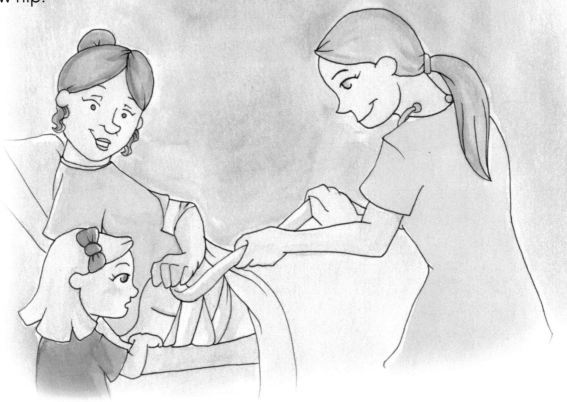

"So when can you come play with me and take me to the park?" asked Taylor.

"Well, my <u>recovery</u> time is about three months, depending on what my doctor tells me. I have to do my exercises every day in order for my hip to get better. My new hip will need some help for about one month, so I will use what are called <u>crutches</u> or a <u>walker</u> when I walk. Then I will be able to walk using a cane for another few weeks. However, there are lots of things we can still do together, such as read books, color, and put together puzzles! Once my boo-boo is all healed, then I will have what is called a <u>scar</u>, which shows where my boo-boo was, but it won't hurt anymore," explained Grandma.

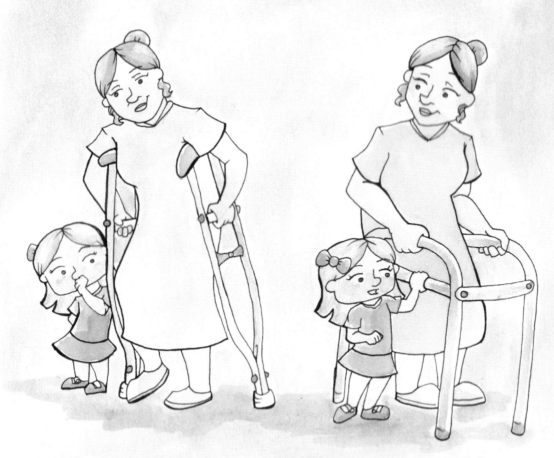

Ashley changed Grandma's bandage and finished up. "Well, my job is done for now," she said. "Taylor, I brought you a little ice cream treat since you are being such a good girl—if it is ok with your mommy."

"Sure, Ashley," said Mommy. "That is very kind of you."

"Yummy!" said Taylor. "I love ice cream! Thank you very much, Ashley. You are very nice."

"It was very nice to meet you Taylor," said Ashley. "When your grandma can come home, make sure to take really good care of her!"

"I will. Thanks again for the ice cream!" said Taylor, as the nurse left the room.

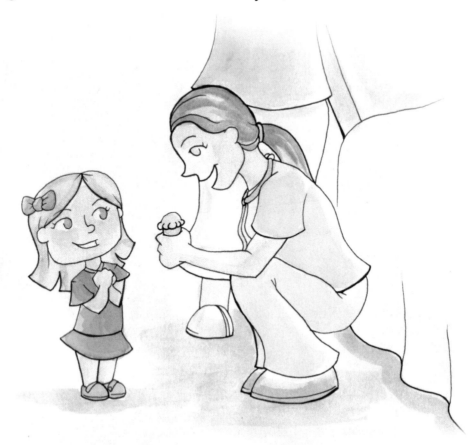

"Can you pick me up, Grandma?" asked Taylor.

"I would love to, Taylor, but I can't do that for a while, because the doctors and nurses told me not to so I don't hurt my new hip. Since I can't pick you up, would you like to come sit next to me on the bed?"

"Yes, please!" said Taylor excitedly. "Why did your hip hurt, Grandma?"

"Well, there are many reasons why people get total hip replacements, but one of the main reasons my hip hurt was because of something called <u>arthritis</u>.

"What is r-thr-eye-tis?" asked Taylor.

"Arthritis is when the cushion between the bones of my hip joint wears out and my bones rub together when I walk," explained Grandma.

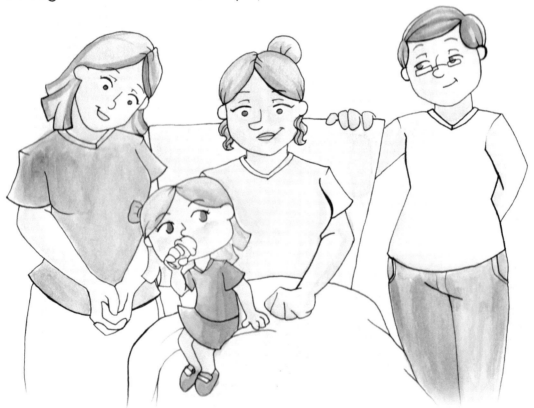

"I am going to show you some pictures of the bones in my hip," said Grandma. "They are called <u>X-rays</u>. The doctor took pictures of my hip bones before and after he put in my new hip.

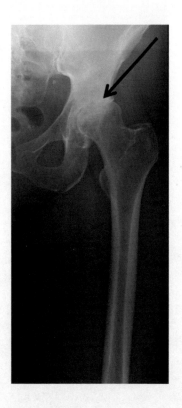

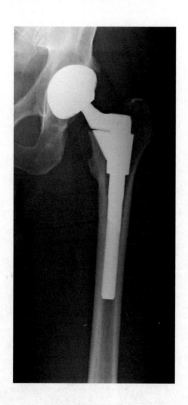

"Here is a picture of my hip before I had surgery. The cushion between my bones has worn away, and that is why I couldn't play at the park with you."

"Is that what you call arthritis?" asked Taylor.

"That is exactly right," said Grandma.

"This is a picture of my hip replacement after my surgery. Now my bones do not rub together, and my hip doesn't hurt anymore. So, now we can go play at the park together."

"Those pictures are really neat, Grandma! Now I know what a hip actually looks like inside our body!"

"Okay, Taylor," said Mommy, "Grandma needs her rest. We can go over to her house when she comes home from the hospital."

"I will come over any time you want, Grandma, and help take care of you. We will still have a great time together while your boo-boo gets better. Maybe Mommy and I will bring cookies next time! How does that sound?"

"That's sounds great," said Grandma.

"I love you, Grandma," said Taylor.

"I love you too," said Grandma.

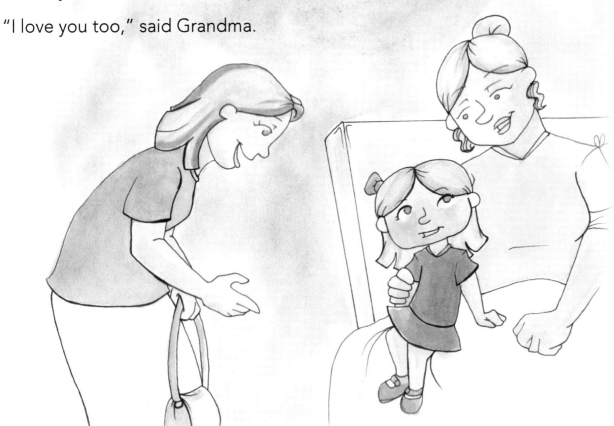

LaVergne, TN USA
19 February 2010
173617LV00003B